BE LAZY,
BURN FAT!!

Table of contents

Ch1
Intermittent Fasting
Timing is key

There are a variety of timing schemes for intermittent fasting, but I personally use "16/8." It's the most efficient for people who train heavy, and it's the most convenient to work around most schedules, but everybody is different. So what is 16/8 intermittent fasting? It's basically just not eating or drinking any calories for 16 hours, sleep included, and utilizing the remaining 8 hours of the day to get all of your calories in. This results in increased fat oxidation, aka fat burn.

Why does this work?

There's a bunch of sciencey stuff behind it, but the meat and potatoes of it is this:

We operate just like a car; movement requires fuel. The difference is, we don't spill over when we fill our tank past capacity. We get fat.

What does the AVERAGE person (not everybody) do on a daily basis?

-They wake up, (for this example, we'll use a 7am wake up time) fuel up the tank with breakfast.

-Go to school /work, (8am) do basically nothing physically.

-Eat a snack. Fuel. (9am-10am ish)

-Take a lunch break, (12pm) , 30 minutes to an hour. Fuel up again.

-Go back to sitting at their desk.

-Leave for the day and go home. (5pm)

-Get/cook dinner. Fuel up again. (6pm-8pm ish)

-Sit on the couch and watch TV.

-Snack. Fuel up, again...(10pm) go to bed.

They spend all day filling the tank, and leave almost no time to burn the gas!

Let's examine the same day, but on a 16/8 intermittent fasting schedule, and without any other dietary change:

-Wake up, (7am)

-Go to school/work at 8am, drinking only water, black coffee, or unsweet tea.

-Go to lunch (12pm) nothing but water, black coffee, or unsweet tea. 30 minutes to an hour to fuck off, read a book, catch up on work, quick workout, etc.

   Note: working out is NOT required. I'm only suggesting that if you already workout to some extent, to utilize the fasting period to get that done. This way, the energy you burn during the workout, as well as the calories burned by the EPOC effect (see: CH.4) work synergistically with your intermittent fasting fat burn.

-Break your fast with a snack. (2pm-3pm ish)

-Leave for the day and go home. (5pm)

-Get /cook dinner. (6-8pm ish)

-Snack (10pm) and goes to bed.

With the 16/8 IF schedule focused around your work day, your daily activities burn off the excess fuel you put in the day before. Then when you start fueling, you have fewer hours before bedtime to cram in your food. You will end up eating less overall, assuming you keep the same bedtime. There's a lot more to it as to WHY you burn more fat, feel an increase in strength, and attain better mental focus/clarity once you adapt to intermittent fasting, but if you understand the fuel analogy, you understand enough to make it work for you.

FAQ's

"Won't I just eat more when I get home?"

You might feel like you're eating more at once, but you'll be eating less overall. If you tried to eat the exact same foods you would always eat, in the exact same quantities, I can almost guarantee that you won't finish it all before bedtime. In fact, the "feast" you can have will leave you so full, your inner fat kid will be DELIGHTED to wait all day for it! Ok maybe that's just me idk. But trust me, it's great.

It's important to note that you will feel much fuller, and stay full for much longer, if you eat real, whole, single-ingredient foods. Another advantage of eating unprocessed foods, is the fact that they are less calorie dense, due to the lack of added fats and sugars. What this means for you, is that you can eat a higher volume of natural food than processed food, to consume the same amount of calories. Pig out on rice, meats, fish, veggies, oats, etc and you'll see what I mean.

"I heard eating before bed is bad, shouldn't I avoid doing that?"

Sure, if you want to. Every body is different, and if you personally find that yours has put on fat the morning after you ate before bed, you're probably right. However I, and many I've trained, routinely fuel up for recovery (sleep) and the next day's activities just before bed, and we stay pretty lean. You should however, avoid SUGAR before bed. Yes, even "natural" sugars from fruit.

"Won't I be hungry all day?"

Yes and no. During the 16 hour fasting period, you're allowed water, BLACK coffee, UNSWEET tea, water, and WATER. 0 calories other than maybe a scoop of amino acids, intra or post workout. (Again, only if this applies to you)

This will do two things:

1- keep you hydrated, since you probably don't drink enough water at the time of reading this.
And 2- keep something in your stomach to push off hunger.

Added bonus: the caffeine from the black coffee/unsweet tea will suppress hunger even further.

Disclaimer: YOU WILL STILL BE HUNGRY AF at the beginning. But I promise, your body will adapt to the new schedule soon, and it will stop sending you those intense hunger signals that you've programmed in by constantly feeding it. Getting through the initial few days or week of adaptation is by far the hardest and only negative aspect of intermittent fasting, other than sometimes you can't squeeze in enough food before bed.

Yeah, you read that right.

That's a serious problem I face, and you might too. One day you'll be so full that you're ready to pop, but check your calorie log for the day and still be 1200 shy of your target, with 30 minutes left to eat. Anyways, if you can get past that initial hunger, the chance of you sticking to it and keeping fat off your body drastically increases. It's by far the hardest part, but thankfully the shortest.

To clarify, you're NOT dropping your calories down to something unsustainable. Some "diets" promote "burning fat fast" by essentially starving yourself.

THIS is not THAT. You're going to FEEL like you're starving, for a few hours a day, until you get home and stuff your face. Once your body adjusts to the new schedule, it'll stop freaking out and telling you to find food all morning.

If only there was a magic pill that could make that transition easy. A supplement that could curb your appetite for a few hours. Something that could burn fat, give you a little energy boost, AND help you focus.

Ch2
EC STACK /FAT BURNER

"The magic pill"

This is a supplement that will curb your appetite for a few hours. It burns fat, gives you a little energy boost, preserves muscle, AND helps you focus.

Seriously. I love this stuff. I take it every year, for 3 months, while I'm focusing on fat loss. Its invaluable to my fat loss regimen.

One more time, just in case a dog chewed up your page one: I'M NOT A DOCTOR. PLEASE CONSULT A LICENSED PHYSICIAN BEFORE ATTEMPTING THIS, OR ANYTHING IN THIS BOOK.

AND DOUBLE YOUR DAILY WATER INTAKE to keep those kidneys good and clear. A good hydration indicator is, to be frank, having clear urine. If it's not clear(-ish) then go knock back a glass of water or two.

So what is the EC stack?

25mg "E" (Ephedrine) +
200mg "C" (Caffeine.)

Some people take it 2-3 times a day, 4 to 6 hours apart. TAKE NO MORE THAN 3 doses a day. Start slow. Don't move up to two doses until you notice that your body develops a tolerance. I only take one dose a day myself, otherwise I won't even think about food until well into my eating window. Take your first dose at 8am, or your equivalent "start of day."

Find your own method of obtaining these (I use bronkaid for my E and caffeine pills for my C) but they're rarely found in the same product anymore, here in the US. Some people advise to add aspirin (making it ECA stack) but I highly advise against it. It complicates things and isn't really necessary. E and C are both pretty solid fat burners individually, but when taken together or "stacked," they work synergistically to achieve a much higher level of fat burn. The EC stack actually causes your body to prioritize fat oxidation as a secondary fuel system (after the glycogen/carbs in your system are burned off) as opposed to the body's default emergency energy source, amino (muscle) breakdown. So in layman's terms, it keeps the muscle tissue you already have, weight-trained or not, and burns off fat, FIRST!

If you decide the EC stack is not right for you, don't worry. You're not alone, and your worries aren't unfounded. There have been cases where people don't obey the rules given, take too much, do a bunch of cardio, and having a heart attack. If your bad at following directions, but you still want to get some extra fat burn going, try a normal retail fat burner from your local store. Similar effect, but they contain far too many chemicals and unknown variables for my liking.

Fat burners, and why they don't work (for most people)

People often think that dietary fat equals fat on their body. They also think that fat burners will burn that same fat if they take it with their food. Neither of these are accurate.

Fat burners keep your hunger at bay, and boost your metabolism. That's it. There's nothing special about them, and they absolutely will not work for anything else than those two things. Sometimes they can give you energy and focus similar to the EC stack, but they will not just melt fat off your body like in the commercials. Most people who take them, don't know how to TIME them for optimal results.

When timed like the EC stack, they work great in conjunction with intermittent fasting. I can't speak on their ability to preserve muscle tissue and prioritize fat burn, but they absolutely keep hunger at bay and ramp up your metabolism for a few hours.

Ch3
MACROS/TDEE

"Getting abs is 20% workouts, 80% nutrition."
"Abs are made in the kitchen."

Ask a typical gym-bro about getting abs, and you're bound to hear one of those two nuggets of wisdom. Despite the fact that most "bro speak" is based on nothing besides "my friend told me this and he's pretty buff," THIS is actually sound advice. This holds true for more than just abs though. It really applies to fat loss in general.

This might feel a little overwhelming at first, but after a while of tracking your macros, you can kinda do it in your head...just keep yourself honest, and use a food scale and a food tracking app every now and then to keep your estimations calibrated.

What are "macros?"

There are three macros (macronutrients): protein, carbs, and fat. These make up every calorie, in every food, that you've ever eaten or ever will eat in your entire life. Therefore it only makes sense to familiarize yourself with them and get them to work for you, instead of keeping you soft and pudgy.

I could go on about macros for days and barely scratch the surface of all there is to know about them. But here's what you need to know to understand them, and to gauge how many of each you should be eating.

• Protein has 4-5 calories per gram.
Proteins are the building blocks that make up muscle (or most any) tissue in the body. It is ESSENTIAL. It keeps you feeling fuller, longer. It also costs the body more calories to process protein, than either of the other macros.

•Carbs have 4-5 calories per gram.
Carbohydrates are energy, plain and simple. They undergo a process called glycogenesis through which they become GLYCOGEN, or ready-to-use fuel for your muscles. SUGARS DO NOT BECOME GLYCOGEN. THEY'RE EITHER IMMEDIATELY BURNED, OR STORED AS BODY FAT. Avoid sugars unless you plan a vigorous workout within 45 (I do 20) minutes of eating it.

• Fat has 9-10 calories per gram.

Fats are not bad, and they certainly do not equate to body fat. We need them, as some of them are ESSENTIAL. They contribute to hormone production, body oils, parts of your skin and nails, and a variety of other things. A fat deficiency can cause hormone imbalances, body system shutdowns, even a decrease in brain health. There are good fats, and there are bad fats. Avoid SATURATED and TRANS FATS if you care about your health. Eat nuts, avocado, fish, and lean meats to get your daily fats. Take fish oil.

Daily macro targets for optimum efficiency will vary from person to person, but here's a good jumping off point that you can tweak after a few weeks to fine tune your progress.

Protein - consume 1g per pound of lean body mass. Some people who exercise intensively (myself included) consume 1g per lb of total body weight. This yields a slightly higher protein intake, leaving less room for fat and carbs.

Fat - consume .4g per pound of body weight. Don't go too much lower than this, or you're just begging for other health issues. Eat "good fats."

Carbs - fill in the rest of your calories with carbs. Dial them back after a few weeks if you're not seeing fat loss. Technically, you could, not count grams of FIBER (like veggies) as carbs for the day, as they do not get utilized. Subtract them from the total carbs if you wish, but I like to overestimate my carb intake by at least that little buffer. That's just me, and people who like to err on the side of lean.

Write down everything you eat, and the caloric values, and the macros. Yes, all the other nutritional info is important, but this book is written strictly from a physique standpoint. The easiest way I found is to download a food tracking app. Remember, this is the lazy way of doing things...but lazy just means more efficient. I personally use My Fitness Pal. (I have no affiliation, I just love the app.) For me, the free version is sufficient, and you can literally enter your food while you eat, in like 1 or 2 minutes. It lets you scan the barcode of any food item and automatically pulls the nutrition info into your daily entry. You can even enter your own foods if you don't find your specific food on the app already. Eat whatever food items you like, so long as they fit in your daily macronutrient budget.

 Remember, IIFYM. If It Fits Your Macros...you can eat it.

TDEE

Total Daily Energy Expenditure. This is the total number of calories that you will burn on a day to day basis, including any physical activities you do. Going to work, lifting weights, breathing, digesting food, and reading this book are all factored in to your TDEE.

Your Basal Metabolic Rate (BMR) is the base number of calories your body burns without accounting for any movement whatsoever. The more muscle tissue you develop, the higher this climbs. BMR is one of a few factors in calculating your TDEE.

To lose weight, all you need to do is this one thing: eat below your TDEE.

FAQ's

"How many calories should I eat?"

There are far too many variables that factor in for me to give a blanket estimate. Google a TDEE calculator and plug in all your personal information (age, height and weight, body fat% activity level etc) or I do offer

personal nutrition consultations at
rdcalvino91@hotmail.com. Of course, each one is
custom to YOU and YOUR body, so I'll still need all
that info.

"What about vitamins?"

Vitamins (or micronutrients) are ESSENTIAL, but I'm
not discussing vitamins other than to say this: we
operate at optimum levels when they are at optimum
levels. A multivitamin a day will keep you from
developing a deficiency. You CAN overdose on the
fat soluble vitamins, A, D, E, and K, so be careful
with those.

"Can I really eat ANYTHING I want?"

Yes, as long as you do not exceed your daily
macronutrient targets. If you blow your entire days
carb and fat budget on pizza cake and ice cream,
you will need to eat basically JUST protein for the
rest of the day. So like, dry tuna. Yum.

Ch4
Workout (optional)
Stack your advantages, multiply your results!

Now up until this point, nothing time consuming has been added to your daily activities, other than the initial download and set-up of an app. If you already worked out before, add this to your toolbox. If not, this is a good starting point. But to emphasize, you do not NEED to workout, to burn fat. Sure it helps speed up your fat loss and keeps your existing muscle tissue from burning off since your body "uses" it on a regular basis, but if you're looking for the easiest, laziest way possible, skip this chapter.

Why workout?

Just like nutrition, I could write for DAYS on the benefits of working out, fasted training, about how to workout for specific goals, body types, target heart rate zones using your VO2 max, and all that sciencey fitness stuff. But in the interest of keeping this short and sweet, ima just throw some bullet points at you and then give you a simple at-home workout routine with built in progression to keep yourself challenged.

• Resistance training beats long, steady state "cardio" hands down, point-blank, period.

• Circuit training (super-sets, giant-sets, etc) is the optimal style of workout to achieve amazing cardiovascular benefits without doing "cardio."

• If you WANT to do cardio, 5 minutes of intense interval "conditioning" burns more fat, is more beneficial, and is less hard on your joints (but waaay harder on your mind) than 30 minutes of steady state cardio. Do conditioning workouts a few times a week and you'll see how much faster your body will change, both visually, and in stamina.

• Fasted training (of any type) will not only give you a more intense workout (because of hormone boosts) but accelerates fat loss by ramping up your metabolism while it's burning away yesterday's excess fuel (body fat.) If you work out during your fasting period, make sure to take one scoop of branched chain amino acids (less than 50 calories worth) to prevent muscle catabolism (breakdown) during your workout.

• 45 minutes of FASTED STEADY STATE cardio (medium effort...you should work for a good sweat) or only 4 - 10 minutes of FASTED CONDITIONING, first thing in the morning EVERY DAY will do WONDERS for steady fat loss.

• Even if you're not following a well-structured workout plan, as long as you work out with INTENSITY, a portion of your calories will be burned off during the workout (obviously) but also AFTER the workout, in what's called Excess Post-exercise Oxygen Consumption. This is basically your body trying to return to its normal (unstressed) state by using oxygen to clear out the lactic acid that built up in your muscle tissue during the workout. There's a lot more sciencey stuff behind it, but suffice it to say that it's basically a caloric "afterburn."

• You'll allocate a portion of the days calories for recovery (you burn calories in your sleep, as your body repairs muscle tissue)

• As you build muscle tissue, your body requires more fuel just to exist (higher BMR = higher TDEE = MORE FOOD)

• Since not everyone has access to gym equipment, I'm sharing a zero equipment (therefore zero excuses) bodyweight workout routine you can do at home, in a hotel, in a garage, elevator, etc

This will test you. It will test your dedication, your will, your creativity, your physical strength, as well as mental. You'll go days or weeks with almost nothing to show for it. You might wanna give up, wondering, "how long until I SEE RESULTS?!"

Well, here's the cheat sheet (assuming you're following ALL the advice in the book so far, you're drinking plenty of water, and you PUSH yourself during these exercises)

3 weeks - POOR results
5 weeks - mediocre results
8 weeks - average results, but notable
3 months - leaner than most
5 months - shredded af, probably the leanest person in the room at most places you go.

RULES

-TAKE A "BEFORE" PICTURE. Not for me to ask you later if I can use it for a testimonial to show the world the amazing results you'll experience, (side note: my email is rdcalvino91@hotmail.com in case you were so blown away by your results that you wanted to let me use them for a testimonial) BUT so that you can SEE the slow, steady progress that you make over time.

These changes happen VERY slowly, each and every day. Especially on your rest days, so mind your nutrition on those "days off." Keep in mind, even poor results are still results, but you won't SEE them without the "before" picture for reference.

-For OPTIMAL results, do THIS 3-5 days a week.

-Do NO LESS than 3 rounds with NO REST in between exercises. Rest NO MORE than 3 minutes (aim for 2) between rounds, if needed. The closer you get to not needing rest, the more of a beast your body will resemble.

-Log your workouts. Track the numbers you hit, and push those numbers up over time. Do more reps, for more rounds. Throw in some burnout sets (sets to muscle failure) on the last round. Take shorter rest periods. You look better when your numbers look better. When you work your way up to 100 pushups in one set, you'll damn well look like it.

-If you can't hit the basic reps for an exercise (I couldn't even do 5 proper pushups back when I was fat) start with an easier variation like wall or knee pushups, door knob pullups, etc., until you can complete at least 10 reps, THEN try the standard version. Once you work up to 20 reps of the standard version, get creative and try a harder version. Trust me, you'll surprise yourself one day.

Here it is. Short and sweet.

-Alternating lunge hops 15/leg (count to 30)
　　　- Start in lunge position, hop up, switch legs and land in lunge position on other foot, repeat.

-15 mid side side crunch (5/5/5)
　　　- 5 standard crunches, and then five crunches laying on either side.

-10 pushups
　　　- Get on your belly and toes and push the earth down with your hands keeping a straight (neutral) spine and tight core, engaged as if you are anticipating a gut punch.

-50 mountain climbers (25/leg) AS FAST AS POSSIBLE
　　　- Just youtube this. Idk how to explain it without demonstration, but i'll give it a shot: get in the "up" position of a

pushup, then bring one knee up to your chest. Quickly alternate legs, keeping your core tight as if you were anticipating a gut punch.

-10 pull ups. Use a towel over a tree branch, rope around a door handle, sheet off a bunk bed, rafter in the garage, etc. Get creative, but ALWAYS be safe and test the weight bearing capacity of whatever your pulling on, SLOWLY. Don't assume anything will hold your full weight all at once. Just find something you can hang onto.

     -FIRMLY GRASP IT, pull yourself up.

-30 second plank. On the last round, hold it for MAX time. Try to increase your max time each workout.

     - Get on your hands or elbows, and your toes. Hold a straight line from head to heels.

FAQ's

"I don't have TIME for an effective workout"

Ok, do you have LITERALLY 4 minutes?

"TABATA"

-The worst 4 minutes of your life, but harder.

-4 minutes broken down into segments of effort and rest.

-Works by creating an "oxygen deficit" in your blood/muscles, sending your body's oxygen consumption (the OC in EPOC) through the roof.

EFFORT (20 seconds)
-MAX EFFORT
-100% ABSOLUTELY the MOST reps you can do in 20 seconds.
-Leave NO gas in the tank.

-MAX EFFORT
-MAXIMUM FUCKING EFFORT

Rest (10 seconds)
-Breathe in that sweet, sweet oxygen.
-Visualize your fat cells being incinerated to fuel this hellish nightmare. If it's your first time, enjoy that false sense of confidence. Run with it. You're probably going to think to yourself "oh this isn't THAT bad"

HAAAHAHAHA

Alternate between "effort" and "rest" until your 4 minutes are up, or you die. Whichever happens first. You will have 8 sets all together. It ends on a "rest," so I always say 7 but whatever. You can do this with burpees (my personal favorite,) squats, jump squats, pushups, pullups, jumping jacks, mountain climbers, high-knees, plank-jacks, power clean, front Squat, bench press, pretty much anything. Mix it up, but try to keep it to ONE or TWO different FULL BODY or MULTI-JOINT movements per session, and a MEDIUM weight (if used) that you can bang out 20 reps with. If you're serious about getting results, but seriously lack time, this will work IF and ONLY IF you push yourself to your MAX limit, every. Single. Time.

Note: for faster results, sprinkle it in 2x a day. The first time in a FASTED state, right when u wake up. And once again before bed...if you got the balls.

FAQs continued

"It's too hard"

No, you're too soft. Start somewhere, and progress.

"My ___ hurts"

Be honest with yourself. Is this really something holding you back? Can you work around it? Or will it defeat you on your quest to get the body of your dreams? Make solutions, not excuses. But also probly see a doctor and make sure it's not a real injury. 9/10 times, you're just being a lil bitch.

"Am I doing this right?"

Probably. Do the movements in front of a mirror if possible, or prop your phone up and leave it recording you to watch your form and compare it to a reliable form video source like bodybuilding.com. Don't let it be an excuse to not do the exercise, just look it up and do it. Don't overthink, just, DO.

"How do I burn *this* fat off? I really just wanna tone my (insert body part here)"

THERE IS NO SUCH THING AS "SPOT" BURNING!!

Fat accumulates on your body in an order specific to YOU, based on YOUR genes. Some people get fat in the face first before any other body part. Some people notice a belly first. Some people get almost exclusively thigh fat. Some, tricep. Usually it's a good spread all over but most people's body has a preference of where to store body fat, first. And second, and third, etc.

It will burn off in the opposite order you packed it on. So last on, first to burn. First on, last to burn. It's that simple.

Fat stored for long enough turns into visceral fat, or fat stored deep inside the body, around the organs. This type of fat is extremely hard to burn off, and is often responsible for that "beer belly" on an otherwise, not so fat (usually older) person. You're not screwed if you have this type of fat, your results will just take longer to show.

In any case, it probably took months or even years to build the fat, so don't expect to lose it all in a couple weeks. Give it a couple months following all the advice in this book and you'll really see a drastic difference.

That's basically it. Apply these techniques with consistency, and you WILL reap the rewards. Take one week to learn and apply each chapter if you need to. Just know that the sooner you integrate these "autopilot" fat burning principles into your everyday life, the sooner you will see the reflection you want, every time you get in front of a mirror.

Remember that to lose weight, all you need to do is eat below your TDEE.

OR

Raise your TDEE above your caloric intake.

OR

A little bit of both, with a little metabolic manipulation using IF, the EC stack, managing your macronutrients, and incorporating a work out for just a FEW minutes on a FEW days each week. This is by far the easiest and most efficient way to get the lean, shredded body you want.

LOG

Use the next few pages to log your calories/macros, if you can't download a food tracking app. Daily calorie and macro tracking is CRUCIAL to a scientific approach. Don't leave ANYTHING up to chance.

DATE	CALS	FAT	CARBS	PROTEIN

DATE	CALS	FAT	CARBS	PROTEIN

DATE	CALS	FAT	CARBS	PROTEIN

DATE	CALS	FAT	CARBS	PROTEIN

DATE	CALS	FAT	CARBS	PROTEIN

GLOSSARY

METABOLISM - the rate at which your body burns calories. Yes, some people have a "slow" metabolism but that's EASILY fixed over time using intermittent fasting alone. Easier if you add the EC stack. Even easier if you adjust it yourself, by increasing your muscle tissue mass. The more muscle you carry, the more calories you burn just to exist.

INTERMITTENT FASTING (IF) - an eating schedule that alternates between fasting and eating periods. 16/8 is the most common, and for good reason.

EPHEDRINE AND CAFFEINE STACK (EC) - the best fat burner if used properly, but it's not for everyone. CONSULT A PHYSICIAN.

CONDITIONING - a more intense version of cardio where you push a lot closer to 100% effort. Increases YOUR "100%" over time, meaning you get faster/stronger/more explosive. Trains your "fight" in fight-or-flight...how long can you give your ALL?

STEADY STATE CARDIO - bike, treadmill, elliptical, jogging a trail, walking, rowing, zumba, etc. Keeping a good, steady pace throughout the duration of your workout, typically aiming for your target heart rate zone. Trains your "flight" in fight-or-flight...how far away can you run before stopping?

RESISTANCE TRAINING - training against resistance. Usually weights or bands, but sometimes just gravity (think pushups/pullups.) The fastest way to increase overall muscle volume, and therefore metabolism.

GLYCOGEN - a multibranched polysaccharide of glucose that gets stored in your muscles and liver. It is used to power the movement of skeletal muscle tissue. It's basically just fuel, made from carbs.

ESSENTIAL - used to describe something that's not naturally produced in the body. We must get this (whatever it is) from our diet. Example: minerals.

DIET - nowhere did I say to "go on a diet," but I want to put this in here anyways because it's so often misused. Everyone is on a diet, assuming two things: 1- they're alive. And 2- they eat something every so often to stay that way. Some people's diets are composed of whole, single-ingredient foods. Others are composed of packaged, processed, filler materials with some real food sprinkled in. What exactly is a hot fry anyways? They're DELICIOUS but why does it light up and melt like that when lit on fire? Idk. Point is, you need to "clean up your crappy diet," not "go on a diet." "Diets" have endpoints. Good nutrition doesn't have an end point. If you view nutrition as having a finish line, YOU WILL end up soft and unhealthy again after you hit your "goal" and get comfortable, I promise. I've seen it 1000 times. The best "diet advice" - eat for fuel, not for flavor. Your reflection will thank you.

CIRCUIT TRAINING - a style of training that attacks several muscle groups. While muscle group 1 is working, 2 and 3 are resting. While 2 is working, 1 and 3 are resting. While 3 is working, 1 and 2 are resting. This allows you to push your body further you thought possible, since your cardiovascular and respiratory systems will be under constant stress, but each muscle group will feel rested again by its turn in rotation. So instead of 30 minutes of cardio, and 30 minutes of lifting, you can do 45 minutes of both simultaneously, which will save time AND push your limits.

BRANCHED CHAIN AMINO ACIDS (BCAA'S) - proteins are the building blocks of muscle. Amino acids are the building blocks of proteins. They are more rapidly absorbed than protein, and have less calories. Consuming one scoop (or less than 50 calories worth) will keep your muscles "fed" while not affecting your "fasting" during a workout. This further prevents your muscles from being burned off for energy.

Idk what else to put in the glossary. I'm probably overlooking something but if you got any questions, shoot me an email at rdcalvino91@hotmail.com and I will respond. Just put the words "FITNESS QUESTION" in the subject line so I know it's important ☐

Made in the USA
Columbia, SC
12 October 2024

43481735R10024